Mommyfesto

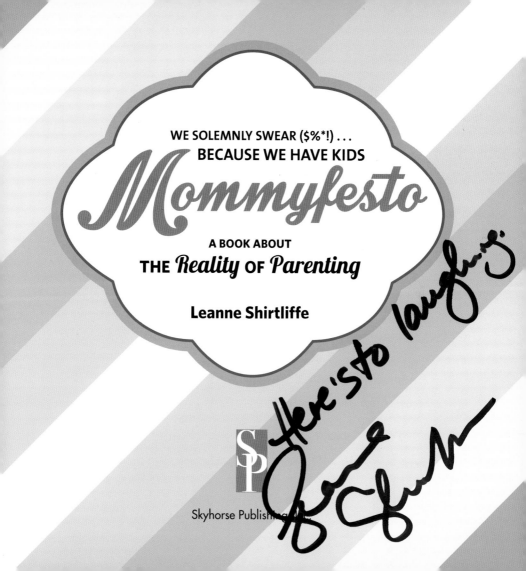

WE SOLEMNLY SWEAR ($%*!) . . .
BECAUSE WE HAVE KIDS

Mommyfesto

A BOOK ABOUT
THE *Reality* OF *Parenting*

Leanne Shirtliffe

Skyhorse Publishing

Here's to laughing.

Skyhorse Publishing books may be purchased in bulk at special discounts for sales promotion, corporate gifts, fund-raising, or educational purposes. Special editions can also be created to specifications. For details, contact the Special Sales Department, Skyhorse Publishing, 307 West 36th Street, 11th Floor, New York, NY 10018 or info@skyhorsepublishing.com.

Skyhorse® and Skyhorse Publishing® are registered trademarks of Skyhorse Publishing, Inc.®, a Delaware corporation.

Visit our website at www.skyhorsepublishing.com.

Select quotes appeared in Leanne Shirtliffe's *Don't Lick the Minivan*, published by Skyhorse Publishing in May 2013 and reprinted with permission.

10 9 8 7 6 5 4 3 2 1

Library of Congress Cataloging-in-Publication Data is available on file.

Cover design by Danielle Ceccolini

Print ISBN: 978-1-62914-696-6
Ebook ISBN: 978-1-63220-051-8

Printed in China

Contents

For Chris. With heaps of love . . . and a bit of sass.

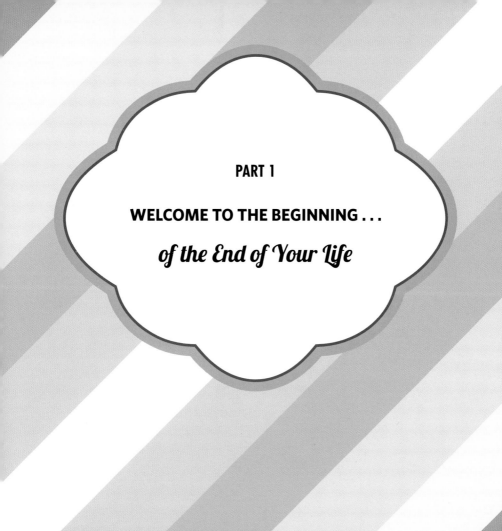

PART 1

WELCOME TO THE BEGINNING . . .

of the End of Your Life

If you can't laugh at yourself, laugh at your kids.

If you can't laugh at your kids, **HIDE IN THE BATHROOM.**

PUTTING YOURSELF IN

TIMEOUT IS A VIABLE

PARENTING STRATEGY.

SO IS MIXING

YOURSELF A MARTINI.

2

The short–term goal of parenting is not to keep the proverbial balls in the air; it's to keep sight of them as they scatter and roll into the gutter.

THE LONG–TERM GOAL OF PARENTING IS TO TRAIN YOUR CHILDREN TO HAVE SLIGHTLY BETTER MANNERS THAN A DOG.

IF IT TAKES A VILLAGE TO RAISE A CHILD, IT'S BEST TO MOVE TO A **SPRAWLING URBAN CENTER.**

HIDING IN THE CLOSET TO HAVE A GOOD CRY OR PLAY ON YOUR SMART PHONE IS AN ACCEPTABLE COPING STRATEGY.

3

The Bermuda Triangle of parenthood is gray hair, wrinkles, and bags under your eyes. Prepare to be lost.

Once You're A Mom, You'll Need A New Makeup Brush. It's Called AN AIR BRUSH.

If guilt burned CALORIES, *no mom would ever need to* DIET.

ON DAYS WHEN RAISING KIDS UTTERLY DEFEATS YOU,

IT'S PERFECTLY NORMAL TO WONDER IF ANGELINA JOLIE WILL

ADOPT YOUR CHILDREN, TOO.

YOU WILL MAKE MULTIPLE MISTAKES AS A PARENT, JUST LIKE WHEN YOU ATTEMPT TO ASSEMBLE A BARBECUE WITH INSTRUCTIONS IN A FOREIGN LANGUAGE.

ONE OF THE MOST OVERLOOKED PARENTING DECISIONS YOU'LL MAKE IS DECIDING WHICH EUPHEMISM TO USE FOR **"FART."**

A MOM WHO SURVIVES THE FIRST YEAR OF PARENTHOOD AUTOMATICALLY GETS A BACHELOR OF SLEEP DEPRIVATION. IF SHE MAKES IT THROUGH THE TERRIBLE TWOS, SHE EARNS A MASTERS IN MARKETING, SPECIALIZING IN FOOD. FINALLY, IF SHE OPTS FOR A SECOND CHILD, SHE'S AWARDED AN HONORARY DOCTORATE IN CONFLICT RESOLUTION, WHICH COMES WITH A FREE PSYCH CONSULT.

You know you're a parent **when half of your daily allotment of energy is spent by 8 a.m.**

Doing laundry, unpacking the dishwasher, and saying "no" are Sisyphean tasks for parents.

The best things in life are free. **EXCEPT CHILDREN.**

A HELPFUL VACATION CHECKLIST:

- ☐ PASSPORTS
- ☐ CLOTHES
- ☐ BOOK
- ☐ KIDS*
- ☐ WINE
- ☐ HUSBAND?

*Ensure kids are 18 or older; if not, stay home.

IF YOU HAVE A

PARENTING MISSION STATEMENT,

YOU NEED A LIFE.

If you're a parent, it's too late.

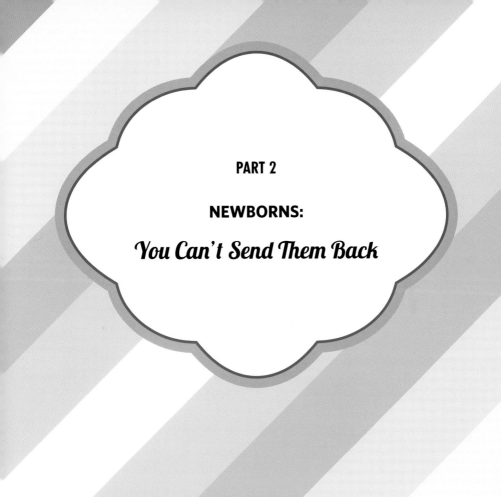

PART 2

NEWBORNS:

You Can't Send Them Back

Every Labor Day weekend, women celebrate that they're not giving birth again.

The term *NATURAL BIRTH* is an oxymoron of moronic proportions.

YOU DON'T LOSE YOURSELF WHEN YOU BECOME **A PARENT**. YOU LOSE YOUR **MONEY**, YOUR **BRAIN CELLS**, AND YOUR **SEX LIFE.**

Swag bags for parents leaving the hospital should include earplugs, a lifetime supply of Band-Aids, and a takeout menu.

HAVING KIDS IS LIKE HAVING HOUSEPLANTS: IF YOU MANAGE TO KEEP THEM ALIVE UNTIL THE NEXT SEASON, YOU'RE A SUCCESS.

THE FONTANELLE IS NOT A TRENDY NEW RESTAURANT WITH **A CANOPY ROOF.**

GIVE YOUR CHILDREN AT LEAST ONE MIDDLE NAME; YOU'LL NEED TO RECITE IT WHEN THEY DON'T LISTEN TO YOU.

Scientists recently revealed that there is DNA related to the Y–chromosome that ensures dads sleep through baby monitor noise.

When you're a parent, the phrase "BEFORE CHILDREN" (B. C.) becomes your version of "ONCE UPON A TIME."

_____

A. D. (AFTER DILATING) becomes your definition of when the craziness starts.

_____

PURCHASING A DIAPER GENIE WILL SAVE YOUR OLFACTORY GLANDS

SO THAT YOU CAN APPRECIATE YOUR BABY'S STALE MILK BREATH.

DADS ARE AN INHERENT PART OF THE PARENTING MARATHON, EVEN BEYOND THAT FLEETING MOMENT WHEN ONE SPERM CROSSES THE FINISH LINE AND COLLAPSES INTO THE ARMS OF AN EGG.

IF YOUR HUSBAND HIRES A BAND TO PLAY FOR YOUR SIX-WEEK CHECKUP, **IT'S NORMAL.**
IF YOU HOPE THE BAND PLAYS LULLABIES, **THAT'S ALSO NORMAL.**

MOTHERING AND PARENTING

SHOULD NOT BE VERBS.

WE ARE MOTHERS.

WE ARE PARENTS.

THAT IS ALL. THAT IS ENOUGH.

SOMETIMES

"MOTHER" TRULY IS THE

ROOT WORD OF

SMOTHER.

BREATHE.

A straightening iron offers a quick fix when you have no time to shower. Avoid using it on unruly leg hair.

Assembling IKEA furniture
blindfolded is easier than
getting a baby into an
INFANT CARRIER.

A uterus looks like an ox skull.
YOU'RE STRONGER THAN
YOU THINK.

Babies frequently laugh at themselves
in the mirror;
tired parents could learn from this.

When your child isn't old enough to fasten her own seatbelt, a drive-thru is your friend. Ensure your local liquor store has one.

MULTITASKING

is cleaning up small milk spills with your socks while holding a baby and texting your therapist.

Delayed breastfeeding: when the Bellagio Fountain comes to a living room near you.

NEW MOMS FREQUENTLY STOP WEARING THEIR SOLITAIRE ENGAGEMENT RINGS BECAUSE THEY LOOK TOO MUCH LIKE PACIFIERS.

Feeding Time: something you thought happened at the zoo. Then you had a baby.

TWITTER AND TEXTING

are good media for new parents, whose brain processing is already limited to 140 characters.

One of the premier events of the Parenting Olympics involves time trials for changing diapers in an airplane bathroom. Difficulty points are awarded if it's done during turbulence.

"HIGH CHAIR" COMES FROM THE LATIN WORD FOR "SLOPPING FOOD ONTO THE FLOOR."

MURPHY'S LAW FOR NEWBORNS: THEY WILL SPEW ONLY WHEN THE BURP CLOTH ISN'T ON YOUR SHOULDER.

TEETHING IS A CONVENIENT EXCUSE TO SLOBBER.

If you're not convinced that **INFANTS ARE CRIMINALS IN DISGUISE,** get their passport photos taken.

IF YOUR BABY LIKES TAKING MEDICINE,
THERE IS NO NEED TO CHUG IT YOURSELF.

REMEMBER WHEN 4:30 A.M. MEANT STAYING UP LATE, AS OPPOSED TO GETTING UP EARLY?

THERE'S A REASON KIDS DON'T COME WITH A MONEY-BACK GUARANTEE: THE LINE FOR RETURNS WOULD BE UNMANAGEABLE.

Cleaning up vomit begins at the end of your
COMFORT ZONE.

WHEN YOU FIND YOUR BABY SUCKING ON THE STROLLER WHEEL IN AN AIRPORT, YOU'RE NOT A NEGLIGENT PARENT. YOU'RE BUILDING UP HIS IMMUNITY.	IF YOU HAVE TIME TO SCRAPBOOK EVERY MOMENT OF YOUR BABY'S LIFE, YOU HAVE TIME TO MAKE AN APPOINTMENT WITH A PSYCHOLOGIST.
THROW YOUR EXPECTATIONS OF CHILDREARING OUT THE WINDOW. IT'S BETTER THAN THROWING OUT YOUR CHILD.	REMEMBER THE GOOD OL' DAYS WHEN CONVERSATIONS (AND BOOKS YOU PURCHASED) DIDN'T INCLUDE BODILY FLUIDS AS A TOPIC?

A PARENT'S SERENITY PRAYER: "GOD GRANT ME THE SERENITY TO ACCEPT THAT I HAVE NO LIFE, THE COURAGE TO LAST UNTIL BEDTIME, AND THE WISDOM TO KNOW WHAT THE HECK I'M SUPPOSED TO BE DOING."

A fully equipped diapering station includes
A HAZMAT SUIT.

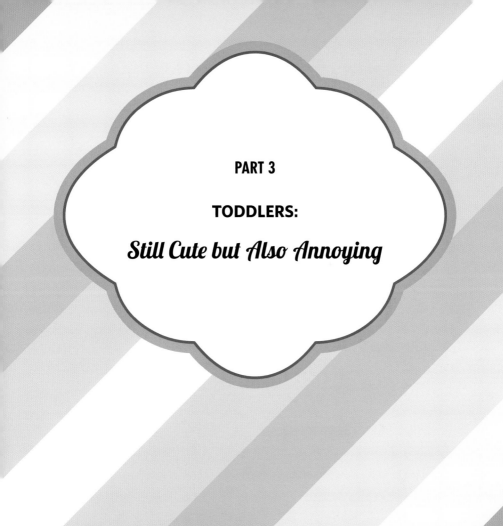

PART 3

TODDLERS:

Still Cute but Also Annoying

Most parents go through more strollers than cars. Payment plans are necessary for both.

The inventor of the vacuum had kids who **PLAYED WITH GLITTER.**

It doesn't help when you blame your child's misbehavior on your partner's genes, **BUT IT'S FUN.**

TELLING YOUR KIDS "MOMMY IS SERIOUS" GIVES YOU THE AUTHORITY OF A GNAT. **SOMETIMES THAT'S ALL YOU NEED.**

16

Convincing your children that the ice cream truck sells only vegetables is fun, even if it puts them on the fast track to therapy.

IT'S NORMAL IF YOUR SON CAN'T REMEMBER TO WIPE HIS OWN BUTT, BUT CAN REMEMBER EVERY LINE OF DIALOGUE FROM GO, DIEGO, GO.

KETCHUP IS A FOOD GROUP. SO IS WINE. THESE TWO FACTS WILL HELP YOU **SURVIVE MANY MEALS.**

IF YOU WANT TO LIVE ON THE EDGE,
WEAR WHITE AND SERVE YOUR KIDS SPAGHETTI.

INTRODUCING NEW FOODS TO YOUR TODDLER REQUIRES THE SKILLS OF A BOMB-DISPOSAL TECHNICIAN AND A TURKEY-STUFFER.

Projectile puke is the only bodily fluid that can be seen from the International Space Station.

MEAL is an acronym for
Mom
Eats,
Always
Last.

The easiest game to play with children is HIDE AND SEEK, *especially if you* "FORGET" TO SEEK.

JEOPARDY NEEDS TO HAVE MOM WEEK.

ANSWERS WOULD INCLUDE "THE PLACE YOUR CHILD LEFT HER FAVORITE STUFFED ANIMAL" AND "THE LAST NIGHT YOU SLEPT MORE THAN FOUR CONSECUTIVE HOURS."

PARKING YOURSELF ON A BENCH AT THE PLAYGROUND TEACHES YOUR KIDS INDEPENDENCE.

ONE OF THE TOUGHEST DECISIONS PARENTS MAKE IS WHETHER TO **SAVE FOR COLLEGE** OR **HIRE A BABYSITTER** AND GO FOR DINNER AND A MOVIE ON A SATURDAY NIGHT.

WHEN YOUR DAUGHTER SAYS THINGS LIKE "ME DO IT," IT MEANS SHE SHARES DNA WITH JAR JAR BINKS AND YODA.

WHEN YOU'VE READ THE SAME BOOK TO YOUR CHILD **42** TIMES, IT'S OKAY TO SKIP PAGES.

Things parents step on, listed by frequency: LEGO, Cheerios, Kids.

When your child is three years old, the alphabet ends: T, U, V, W, X, WHY, WHY, WHY?

Play dates: a legitimate reason for moms to start drinking at noon.

The person who said, "The less you give a damn, the happier you will be" **NEVER LEFT A TODDLER IN A ROOM WITH A MARKER.**

Hosting a birthday party for a child is supposed to be painful. It reminds you of what giving birth was like.

KIDS DON'T LIKE GREEN VEGETABLES OR MUSTARD

because these foods are the colors of their baby sibling's poo.

PARENT HACK 1: CAR SEATS AND SEATBELTS HELP YOU TRANSPORT BOTTLES OF WINE HOME SAFELY.

PARENT HACK 2: SEW MOP HEADS TO YOUR CRAWLING CHILD'S KNEES.

PARENT HACK 3: SIPPY CUPS DOUBLE FOR WINE TRAVEL CUPS AT THE SOCCER FIELD.

PARENT HACK 4: SPRAYING WINDEX ON EXORCIST-TYPE PUKE STAINS REMOVES THE STENCH. SPRAYING IT ON YOUR BABY IS LESS EFFECTIVE.

PARENT HACK 5: PARK OUTSIDE A STORE WITH FREE WIFI WHEN YOUR CHILD IS SLEEPING IN HIS CAR SEAT.

POTTY TRAINING IS LIKE BEING REALLY DRUNK:

You spend a lot of time peering into the toilet bowl and swear if you get through this you'll never do it again.

INVESTING IN AN OUCH-LESS
BRUSH WILL
SAVE YOUR RELATIONSHIP
WITH YOUR DAUGHTER.

WHEN YOU HAVE CHILDREN,
"FINE DINING" MEANS
CRAYONS, KIDS MENUS,
AND BEIGE FOOD.

THE VOMIT FAIRY IS AN EVIL, ACID-HEADED ALIEN.

A child who will not fall asleep puts
THE RUM IN "GRUMPY."

IT'S OKAY TO
UNFRIEND PEOPLE WHO
BRAG ABOUT WHAT HEIGHT
PERCENTILE THEIR CHILD IS IN.

IT'S MANDATORY
TO UNFRIEND PEOPLE WHO
BRAG ABOUT HOW GIFTED
THEIR CHILD IS.

Childless Relatives:

FAMILY EXPERTS ON HOW TO RAISE KIDS PROPERLY.

WHEN YOUR CHILD STARTS SPEAKING IN FULL SENTENCES, EVERY DAY IS NON SEQUITUR DAY.	CHILDFREE WOMEN: THOSE WHO GET TO EAT A MEAL WHILE IT'S STILL WARM.
WHEN YOU DON'T HAVE TIME TO SHOWER, TAKE SOLACE IN THE FACT THAT MANY EXHAUSTED MOMS ARE ROCKING THE FRENCH DIRT MANICURE.	YOU KNOW YOU'RE THE MOTHER OF A TODDLER WHEN YOU POUR YOUR GUESTS A CUP OF COFFEE THAT IS ONLY HALF FULL.

MONDAY (THE DAY THAT'S THE GUTTER OF THE WEEK) BEARS AN UNCANNY RESEMBLANCE TO MOM-DAY. JUST LIKE HOW FRIDAY IS REALLY FRIED-DAY.

22

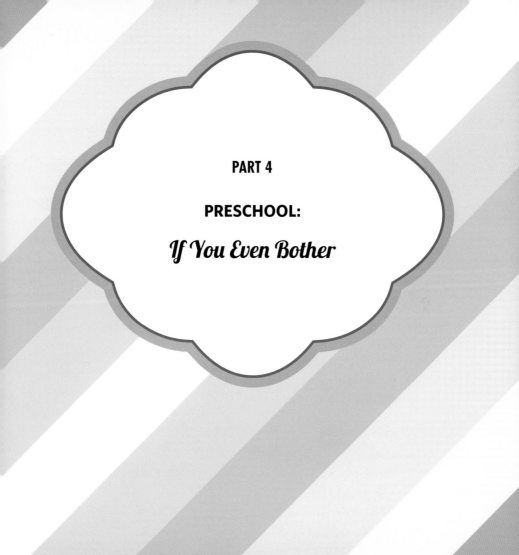

PART 4

PRESCHOOL:

If You Even Bother

A person who is nice to adults but is not nice to kids is called MOM.

A parent's character can be judged by her ability to get the
RATIO OF CHEERIOS TO MILK CORRECT.

Bedtime is a nightly showdown and
YOU'RE OUT OF AMMO.

EVERYTHING THAT'S

WRONG WITH PARENTING

CAN BE FOUND DOWN THE VENT

IN THE PLAYROOM.

If you can survive parented piano lessons, you can survive a zombie apocalypse.

A BAND—AID AND A KISS SOLVE MOST DAILY CRISES.
SO DOES SPEAKING PIRATE.

HOLDING AN AFTER-HOURS FUNERAL FOR YOUR DAUGHTER'S STRIPPER BARBIE IS
GOOD PARENTING.

IF YOUR MINIVAN HAS ENOUGH CRUMBS ON THE FLOOR TO FEED A GAGGLE OF GEESE,
YOU'RE NORMAL.

TRYING TO CONVINCE YOUR CHILD NOT TO LEAVE THE WATER TAP RUNNING PUTS **THE MENTAL IN ENVIRONMENTAL.**

When your child learns to read, her world opens. You, on the other hand, have to learn to focus on *Inner Peace for Dummies* while she provides the sound effects for her book, *Farts from Around the World.*

Eating your kid's Halloween candy helps reduce CHILDHOOD OBESITY.

Taking children to a theme park puts the NOW *in* XANAX.

THE PREQUEL TO *GO THE F**K TO SLEEP* IS *BRUSH YOUR TEETH ALREADY.*

SPRING BREAK SHOULD BE RENAMED SPRING BREAKDOWN.

THE BEST PART OF VACUUMING IS THE SOUND LEGO PIECES MAKE WHEN THEY'RE SUCKED UP.

AN ORGANIZATION WORTHY OF STARTING IS **MASS**: MOTHERS AGAINST SOCCER SEASON.

YOU'VE HOSTED A SUCCESSFUL BIRTHDAY PARTY IF YOU HAVEN'T HAD TO CALL 9-1-1.

If aliens saw a cereal box after a child opened it, they'd conclude he hadn't been fed for weeks.

The sponsor of beginner violin lessons IS VALIUM.

Not wanting to learn how to put your child's hair in a bun is a good reason to keep her out of ballet.

The formative years are sponsored by Play-Doh, which is the short form of PARENTS NO LONGER HAVE ANY <u>DOUGH</u> LEFT FOR PLAY.

The lungs of the average preschool child contain enough glitter for a fairy party.

Nothing reminds you of the relentlessness of childhood like
BOTTLE DRIVES AND BAKE SALES.

ACCEPT THE FACT THAT YOUR HOME WILL MOONLIGHT AS AN ORPHANAGE FOR BROKEN CRAYONS.

When American forefathers fought for the "right to bear arms," they weren't talking about glue guns and pinking shears.

Prepare to debate essential topics with your children, like
WHERE THE HECK MAX AND RUBY'S PARENTS ARE.

HIRING A HIT MAN TO TAKE OUT THE CREATORS OF CARTOON THEME SONGS IS TEMPTING, ALBEIT ILLEGAL.

WHEN YOUR CHILD STARTS SINGING ALONG TO KIDZ BOP COMMERCIALS, IT'S TIME TO LIMIT TV.

HUMILITY: HAVING TO ASK YOUR FOUR-YEAR-OLD HOW TO WORK YOUR TV. AND YOUR SMART PHONE, IF YOU CAN FIND IT.

Don't panic if you have no snacks starting with "J" for your kindergarten child's J–Day celebration. SIMPLY GRAB A SHARPIE AND SEND JOGURT.

EVIL, THY NAME IS WHINING.

MINIATURE PLASTIC DINOSAURS ARE LANDMINES FOUND ON YOUR FLOOR IN THE MIDDLE OF THE NIGHT.

THE BEST THING ABOUT THE MONTH OF DECEMBER IS BEING ABLE TO USE SANTA CLAUS AS A THREAT.

To parent a difficult child,

MOVE CLOSER TO GRANDPARENTS.

INCESSANT TELLING OF KNOCK–KNOCK JOKES MAKES PARENTS WANT TO KNOCK–KNOCK THEIR HEADS AGAINST THE WALL.	IMAGINARY FRIENDS ARE AN IMPORTANT DEVELOPMENTAL MILESTONE FOR CHILDREN. AND FOR MOTHERS MAROONED IN SUBURBIA.
TABLE MANNERS: AS ELUSIVE AS PEACE IN THE MIDDLE EAST.	THE SOUNDTRACK FOR BEDTIME INCLUDES THE THEME FROM *JAWS*.

Little known fact: the alarm clock was invented
by someone who didn't have kids.

PART 5

THE SCHOOL YEARS:

Apparently the Teachers Are Responsible for Them Only Six Hours a Day

Peace on Earth is a lofty goal. Peace in your house is loftier still.

Be weirder than your kids and THEY'LL START TO ACT NORMALLY.

THE BOTTOM OF YOUR CHILD'S **BACKPACK** CONTAINS MORE **DETRITUS** THAN THE FLOOR OF A **MOTÖRHEAD CONCERT.**

32

Boxing Day should be renamed International Pajama Day, or Don't-You-Dare-Complain-That-You're-Bored Day.

HOW-TO-PARENT BOOKS MAKE GREAT PAPERWEIGHTS FOR YOUR CHILD'S ART PROJECTS IN THE RECYCLING BIN.

THE BOOK TITLED *THE PARENTS' GUIDE TO EVERYTHING*
IS FILLED WITH BLANK PAGES.

HIDING IN THE PANTRY TO EAT YOUR HIDDEN STASH OF CHOCOLATE IS SENSIBLE. INSTALLING A LOCK ON THE PANTRY DOOR IS EVEN MORE SENSIBLE.

You know you're a tired mom when your brain is toast and there's no Nutella in sight.

You have a better chance of winning the lottery than having ALL SOCKS MATCH when you're folding laundry.

Once your child can play "BORN TO BE WILD" on the kazoo, your job as a parent is FINISHED.

UNWRAPPING INDIVIDUALLY PACKAGED GRANOLA BARS AND THROWING THEM INTO TUPPERWARE CONTAINERS IS A VIABLE STRATEGY FOR SURVIVING LITTER-LESS LUNCHES IN CELEBRATION OF EARTH WEEK AT YOUR CHILD'S SCHOOL.

ONE OF THE MILESTONES OF HITTING THE TWEEN YEARS IS WHEN YOUR CHILD DISCOVERS MADLIBS . . . AND THE JOY OF USING "BUTT" AS A NOUN.

THE PURPOSE OF SUMMER VACATION: TO MAKE KIDS SO BORED THEY'LL WATCH EDUCATIONAL PROGRAMS ON THEIR OWN.

IF YOU SPEND YOUR FRIDAY SUPERVISING AN ELEMENTARY SCHOOL DANCE, YOU MAY NEED A LACK-OF-SOCIAL-LIFE INTERVENTION.

When your child says, "Why do you need to go on a date? You're married," you've waited too long.

If your brain cells feel like they're moving too slowly, take your kids on rides at an amusement park FOR A DAY.

When your children don't appreciate your imitation of a dot matrix printer, it's proof that the younger generation is lagging behind.

You know your life is over when YOU GO TO BED BEFORE YOUR CHILDREN.

Showing your kids how to smuggle food into movie theaters is a chapter in in the book **TEACHING CHILDREN TO BUDGET.**

The term *peewee hockey* is French for "be prepared to carry more gear than a Sherpa climbing Mount Everest."

BIRTHDAY PARTY LOOT BAGS:
ensuring dollar stores stay in business.

In Sweden, helicopter parents are called "curling parents" because they sweep obstacles out of the way for their kids. And because they're raising future winter Olympians. And because they sometimes say "Hurry! Hard!" in the bedroom.

A Mom's Nine Circles of Hell

1. TV programming for tweens.
2. Kids practicing the recorder.
3. Parents who share clips of their kids practicing the recorder.
4. Children's music that's stuck on repeat play.
5. Children dressed in snowsuits who have to go pee.
6. Parents who say, "Oh, you think this stage is bad? Just wait until they're older."
7. School cancelations.
8. Kids who are sick.
9. Husbands who are sick.

MURPHY'S LAW:
YOUR KIDS WILL WAKE YOU UP
AT 5:30 A.M.
THROUGHOUT THE HOLIDAYS,
BUT SLEEP UNTIL 7:30 A.M.
ON SCHOOL DAYS.

WHEN YOUR TWEENS START
TRADING "YO MAMA" JOKES,
IT'S TIME TO BREAK OUT
THE HARD LIQUOR.
BECAUSE YO MAMA DRINKS
LOTS OF BOURBON.

MATH FOR PARENTS INVOLVES SOLVING FOR ZZZZ.

The algebraic equation for the time that your children need to be asleep (t) before the tooth fairy visits (tF) is

$$\frac{(tF - t)\text{martini}^2}{\$ \text{ in wallet}} = Zzzz$$

JUST BECAUSE YOUR CHILD IS
"GIFTED" DOES NOT MEAN THAT
HE CAN BE RETURNED FOR A
REFUND.

IT'S DIFFICULT TO
EXPLAIN SEX TO A CHILD
WHO STILL WRITES LETTERS
TO SANTA.

38

GAMES NIGHT: reducing children to tears for generations.

BY BEDTIME, MOST MOTHERS FEEL LIKE THEIR KIDS HAVE PLAYED A FEW ROUNDS OF **WHACK-A-MOM.**

WHEN YOUR CHILD STARTS USING COMIC SANS FONT, IT'S TIME TO OUTSOURCE HER PARENTING.

Some days

THE HUNGER GAMES MAKES SENSE.

SCIENCE FAIR PROJECTS: HELPING PARENTS EARN A SOLID B FOR THEIR CHILD.	SARCASM AND HYPERBOLE ARE THE LEFT JAB AND UPPERCUT OF THE SUCCESSFUL PARENT.
SLEEPOVERS ARE LIKE REALITY TV: THEY'RE FASCINATING WHEN THEY OCCUR IN SOMEONE ELSE'S HOUSE.	TALKING TO YOUR DAUGHTER ABOUT MENSTRUATION WITHOUT EVOKING A B-MOVIE MASSACRE SCENE IS DIFFICULT.

TEACHING YOUR CHILDREN ABOUT IRONING IS NOT AS IMPORTANT AS TEACHING THEM ABOUT IRONY.

IRONY:

when lousy parents turn into awesome grandparents.

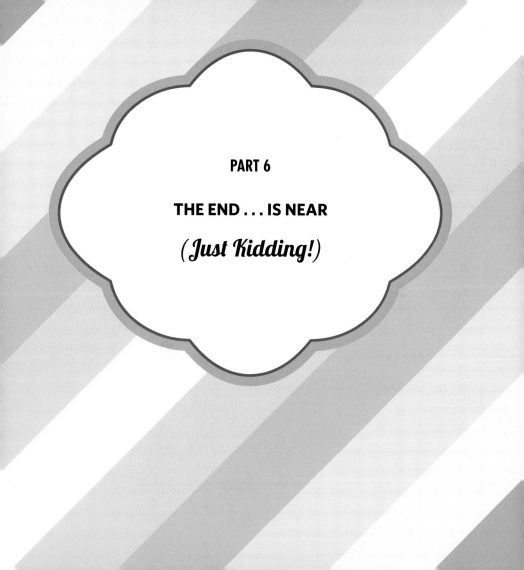

PART 6

THE END . . . IS NEAR

(Just Kidding!)

Some phases of life are harder than others. Like parenting.

If you think you're a bad parent,

WATCH REALITY TV.

IT'S IMPORTANT TO

CELEBRATE THE

SMALL THINGS.

LIKE BEDTIME.

AND SCREW-TOP WINE.

Having a dog is not like having a child. You can't crate a kid, at least not for long.

SAVING FOR THERAPY IS AS ESSENTIAL AS SAVING FOR COLLEGE. AND AS EXPENSIVE.

PINTEREST IS A SOCIAL NETWORK THAT REMINDS YOU THAT YOU SUCK.

IF YOU GOT A DIME EVERY TIME SOMEONE TOLD YOU RAISING KIDS WAS EASY, YOU'D HAVE ONE DIME. MAYBE.

Web MD: Helping
NORMAL
parents become
NEUROTIC.

GMS, OR GUILTY MOTHER SYNDROME,

IS A CONDITION THAT MOMS SUFFER FROM MORE FREQUENTLY THAN PMS

(SEE ALSO WEB MD).

THE FACT THAT MALE SEAHORSES HAVE BABIES IS A GOOD REASON TO BELIEVE IN REINCARNATION.

THE FACT THAT APHIDS ARE BORN PREGNANT IS A GOOD REASON NOT TO BELIEVE IN **REINCARNATION.**

IT'S OKAY TO WATCH A NATURE DOCUMENTARY ON

ANIMALS THAT EAT THEIR YOUNG

TO ASSURE YOURSELF YOU'RE NOT

THE WORST PARENT EVER.

"It's just a stage"
is a good parenting mantra.
So is
"I booked a babysitter."

If parents actually manage
one minute of foreplay,
it involves locking the
bedroom door.

Foreplay is
what you had time
FOR B. C.

DAYLIGHT SAVINGS TIME:

Robbing sleep from parents for generations.

DATE NIGHT:

TWO HOURS THAT REMIND YOU THAT

YOU ACTUALLY LIKE YOUR SPOUSE.

> The phrase WOE ME can be found in "overwhelmed." WINE cannot be found; it's been consumed.

TO KEEP THE BIRTHRATE DOWN AND

PREVENT OVERCROWDING,

GIFT *MOMMYFESTO* TO YOUR FRIENDS.

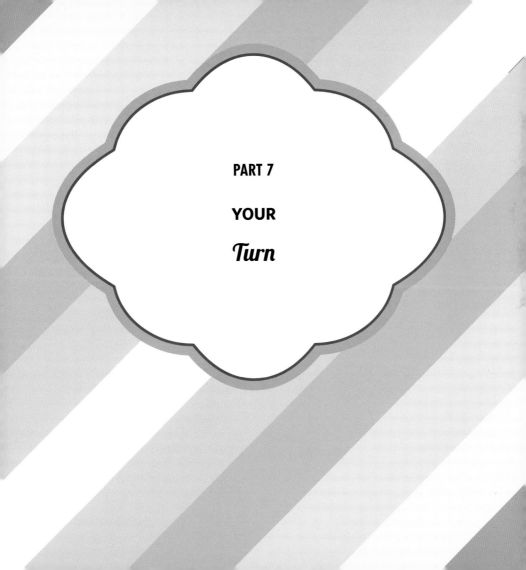

PART 7

YOUR

Turn

Pour yourself a martini and scribble your own Mommyfesto proclamations!

Submit your own Mommyfesto proclamation at IronicMom.com/contact/ for a chance to be featured on Leanne Shirtliffe's blog.

Pour yourself a second martini and scribble your own Mommyfesto proclamations!

Submit your own Mommyfesto proclamation at IronicMom.com/contact/ for a chance to be featured on Leanne Shirtliffe's blog.

Hide from your children and scribble your own Mommyfesto proclamations!

Submit your own Mommyfesto proclamation at IronicMom.com/contact/ for a chance to be featured on Leanne Shirtliffe's blog.

50

Hide in the bathroom and scribble your own Mommyfesto proclamations!

Submit your own Mommyfesto proclamation at IronicMom.com/contact/ for a chance to be featured on Leanne Shirtliffe's blog.

Hire a babysitter and scribble your own Mommyfesto proclamations!

Submit your own Mommyfesto proclamation at IronicMom.com/contact/ for a chance to be featured on Leanne Shirtliffe's blog.

Drop your kids off at a relative's house and scribble your own Mommyfesto proclamations!

Submit your own Mommyfesto proclamation at IronicMom.com/contact/ for a chance to be featured on Leanne Shirtliffe's blog.

Pour yourself a glass of wine and scribble your own Mommyfesto proclamations!

Submit your own Mommyfesto proclamation at IronicMom.com/contact/ for a chance to be featured on Leanne Shirtliffe's blog.

Pour yourself a second glass of wine and scribble your own Mommyfesto proclamations!

Submit your own Mommyfesto proclamation at IronicMom.com/contact/ for a chance to be featured on Leanne Shirtliffe's blog.

55

Acknowledgments

As bizarre as it may seem, this book would not have existed if it weren't for some men in my life. Thanks to Clay Morgan, who insisted that *Mommyfesto* was too good an idea to ignore. Thanks to Brad Somer, who said my draft pages should be a book. My husband Chris somehow manages to support me and to make me laugh ridiculously every darn day. Without him, I wouldn't have had the confidence to trust my humor. My brother, Steve, is a funny man I've always looked up to—and not just because he's tall and loud.

And the women. My housewives: you know who you are. My writing besties: Trish, Elena, Nancy, Erin, and Marianne. Patti, who has to be the proudest big sister ever; it goes both ways, eh? Agent Jill Marr, who is two-parts awesome and one-part superhero. Editor Julie Matysik, who manages to be encouraging and constructive at the same time and who magically answers emails the day I send them.

And my parents: Jim and Janice, who gave me the basic needs: food, shelter, and sarcasm. And that unconditional love thing, too.

And Calgary: a city that embraces me and my humor, and makes me feel that this is my home (except for the fact I still cheer for the Winnipeg Jets).

Finally, for Vivian and William, the two funniest ten year olds I know. I'm glad you chose me to be your mom. Now go to bed. And please sleep past 5:30 a.m.